MOOD SWINGS

HOW TO CONTROL YOUR MOOD SWINGS TO AVOID EMOTIONAL ROLLERCOASTER'S

By Patricia A. Carlisle

Introduction

I want to thank you and congratulate you for choosing the book, *"MOOD SWINGS: How to avoid mood swings to avoid Emotional Rollercoaster's"*.

This book contains proven steps and strategies on how to avoid mood swings and avoid emotional rollercoaster's.

Have you ever skipped from great mood to terrible, possibly three or four times- notwithstanding, nothing in the real world has changed? A great many individuals take medication to suppress their mood swings. In 2011, drug companies sold $11 billion dollars of antidepressants, antipsychotics, to fight additional weakening tribulations like bipolar issues and mental trips included $18 billion.

At that point, there are millions more who experience the bad effects of sort of mellow yet discomforting feeling of moodiness that prompts terrible choices like offering an underestimated stock or squabbling with your life partner, however it doesn't justify a solution.

Like anything else, mastering your moods takes practice. Whatever routines you pick, move rapidly before the unsettling begins to eat at itself. Get a clear view and understand the situation. There are various psychological twists that makes things appear worse than they truly are, and in this way, trigger terrible moods.

Hence, Greek logician Epictetus' perception: "Individuals are not exasperates by things, but rather by the perspective that they take of them." In this book you will learn to see a different perspective on how you see things and avoid emotional rollercoaster's.

Thanks again for choosing this book, I hope you enjoy it!

Table of Content

Preview Of 'Coping with Anxiety Disorder: How to stop anxiety tension.'

Chapter 1

MOOD SWINGS

A mood swing is just a recognizable change in one's mood or enthusiastic state. Everyone has mood swings, and they are a characteristic piece of a lot of people's lives. We get happy, we get sad, We have a time of feeling like we are on top of the world and in charge, and sometimes, we feel drained, dormant and whipped. Occasional mood swings are a part of the vast majority of our lives.

Unfortunately, for a few individuals' mood swings are so drastic, fast or real; that they interfere with their everyday life. Bipolar is the best sample of an issue that is described by mood swings-from hyper to depress. You cannot withstanding have mood swings between any two feelings, pitiful to furious, cheerful to sad. Let us identify some of the reasons for mood swings in individuals.

Chapter 2

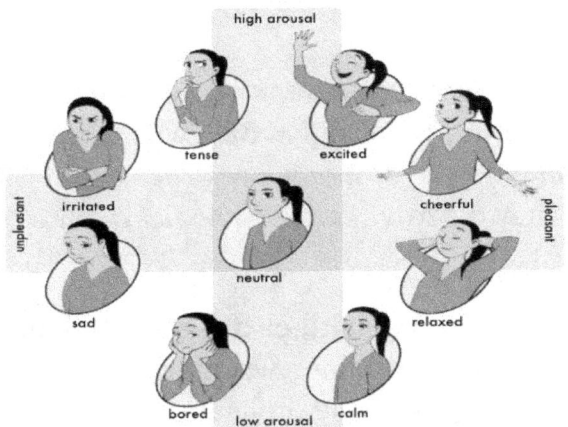

BASIC CAUSE OF MOOD SWINGS

Stress is a critical factor behind mood swings in people. individuals manage stress in different ways. Some handle it better than others. When we have a considerable measures on our plate such as a disagreement with our friends, money related problems, difficult friends or relatives, or what every else, sometimes it can develop into an excessive amount that we can't separate. Not everyone with stress communicates anger. Some discouraged individuals get furious or unsettled. You may not understand that your mood swings are really an indication of stress.

Bipolar issue is thought to be demeaned in the U.S. since patients frequently look for assistance from a specialist when they are depressed, however, not when their mood is forceful. When in the hyper stage, patients have a great amount of energy, and most of the time they do not rest, overspend their funds, or do things excessively such as, paint the whole house in one day. A few individuals can switch between the two extremes.

Rest is super essential. The individuals who don't get enough sleep can become uncontrollable, and have a difficult time managing life stressors.

Alcohol and **illegal drugs,** for example, cocaine and methamphetamines, can bring on a high. But, what goes up must in the long run come down. Not only are drugs awful for our physical wellbeing, they destroy our psychological wellness too.

The vast majority of people can deal with **caffeine** at 1-2 cups a day; However not every, caffeine when drinking at abundance can make you anxious, bring on heart palpitations, and impact mood.

The same goes for **sugar**. It may give you extraordinary energy at the beginning, however when sugar wears off, we have a tendency to crash, and use up the energy that we stored, and thus, our mood plunges.

Also, at times our hormones do have an impact on our mood. Some individuals who experience the bad effects of **PMS** report mood swings up to two weeks preceding the time of their periods. Estrogen withdrawal can take over your mood, as well. When your estrogen levels drop, ladies simply don't feel well. I regularly hear ladies complain about mood swings, depression, and tension when they are encountering this period of their life.

Chapter 3

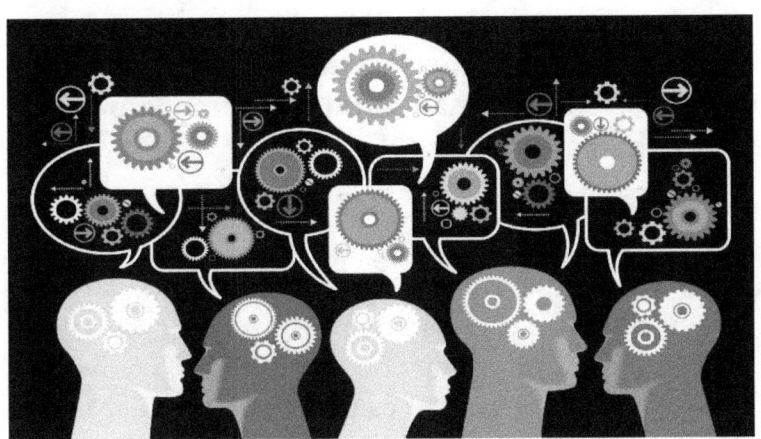

HOW TO CONTROL AND ELIMINATE THE CAUSES OF MOOD SWINGS

Steven Berglas, practicing analyst for a long time and previous clinical educator at the Harvard Medical School, has some expertise in helping top officials and competitors manage stress, burnout and other psychological turmoil, and he's filled with practical advice on holding hurtful instability under wraps.

POLARIZED THINKING

This mental breakdown depicts the tendency to see the world in a highly contrasting way. If you're not manufactured like a NFL linebacker, you're a thin weakling; if you're not a CEO of a multibillion company, you're a useless disappointment. Computers bargain in zeroes and ones, yet people shouldn't. Rather, place things in connection by appointing some unpleasant numbers. Illustration: That last huge deal might fail to work out for instance, yet perhaps you're batting more than .300 for the year.

OVERGENERALIZATION

It's shockingly simple and absolutely unreasonable to think one negative time is a forerunner of disaster. Do you think Tiger Woods ever stressed that an awful golf game implied his entire season was in danger?

FORTUNE TELLER'S ERROR

This emerges when you have no genuine data around important issue-so you fill the void by presuming that no news is terrible news. Let's assume you thought a prospective employee meeting went well, however the organization is taking as much time as required to get back in contact with you. There's no motivation to accept the news is terrible, yet the absence of information is reason for gloom. Prepare for awful news (get caught up with setting up more meetings), yet don't build up an ulcer.

PERSONALIZATION

We want to connect negative acts to irrelevant result "Typhoon Sandy desolated my cellar, so God must have it out for me!"-Lose the self-importance. Keep in mind that you're not the focal point of the universe-and be exceptionally thankful for that.

EXTERNALIZATION

We frequently credit our moods to outside contacts instead of to their actual source. Don't smear basic certainties with false importance. If there's a genuine issue, make the opportunity to take a shot at it.

Chapter 4

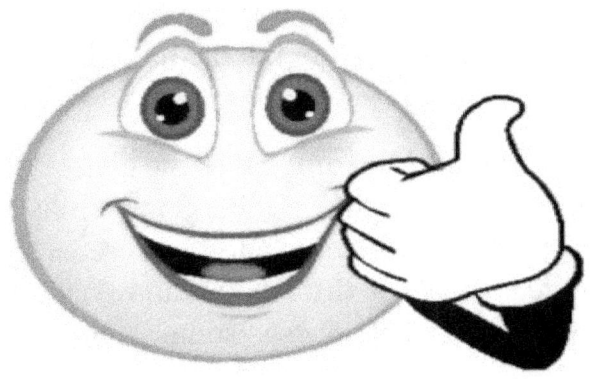

TACTICS TO CONTROL YOUR MOOD SWINGS

Consider what's known as the James-Lange standard of feeling, it was develop by two 19th century clinicians William James and Carl Lange. James and Lange speculated that feelings are reactions to a thought or experience. Case in point: You keep running from a bear because you know it can destroy you. Conclusion: "I'm perplexed about the bear on the grounds that I'm running from it." Exploration has demonstrated that the James-Lange guideline lives up to expectations, as well.

If our bodies move in a particular way, our moods will adjust as need be, contingent upon the connection in which we're moving. One test included two groups of individuals with fake cathodes joined around their lips and chins. With no further clarification, the first group was asked to form a smile, while the second was told to wear a frown. Afterward, the subjects were given funny cartoons while the "anodes" were being "aligned." Result: The individuals already requested that smile helped in enjoying the cartoons more than those who were assigned to frown.

Building on the above findings we can use the tactics below to control our mood swings.

1. Throw your weight around. Heading off to the gym aids, however just to some extent, says Berglas. While discharging endorphins and pressing additional reps can place you in great spirits, awful moods can weaken force and hurt execution so cut yourself some slack.

2. Acting brave on the outside with head high, chest out, and look firm- helps you feel positive and solid within, says Berglas. Balancing out the criticism from other people who through non-verbal prompts, recognize and look upon your quality.

3. Most terrible moods start as "I'll-never-get-there-from-here" self-crushing proclamations. "Great books" you've begun three times however, will never complete; and apparel that will never fit. Not just will your mood lift, you'll have more vitality for the things that truly needs your consideration at this time.

4. Drink less, a few cocktails can settle your nerves, however, not for long, as your body forms the alcohol, disforia and enthusiastic state, that's why nervousness, and an uneasy state soon kicks in.

Chapter 5

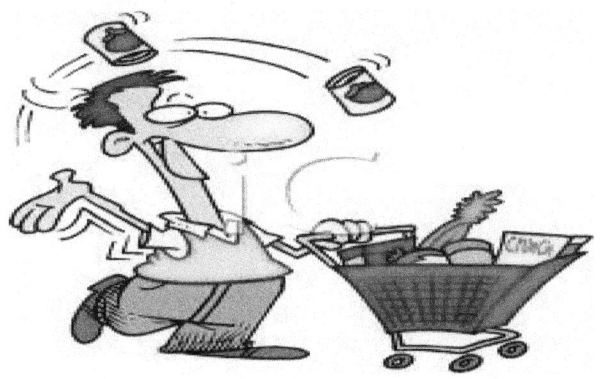

TIPS TO AID IN CONTROLLING YOUR MOOD SWINGS

- Get no less than 8 hours of rest every night, and keep a normal rest wake cycle. Try not to sit in front of the TV, or do anything in bed other than sex and rest.

- Try not to drink more than one cup of coffee a day, or better yet, none by any means, particularly if you are sensitive to caffeine.

- Drugs can genuinely affect how we manage life. They may show you a bit of mercy from your stressors immediately while you're using them; however the aftermath dangers are just not justified.

- Stay away from excessive carbs. Stay on an eating regimen comprising of a complex carbs with protein at every supper, with no less than 5 servings of leafy foods a day.

- Throw away those caffeinated beverages and any beverages with sugar. Drink a lot of water for the duration of the day-add a cut of lemon.

- Whether it's playing a game, joining a yoga class, figuring out how to sew, or anything that interest you, pastimes are extraordinary outlets for our life stressors, and help keep us adjusted.

Keep in mind that if you ever have contemplations of harming yourself, or any other person, you should talk to your doctor immediately.

Chapter 6

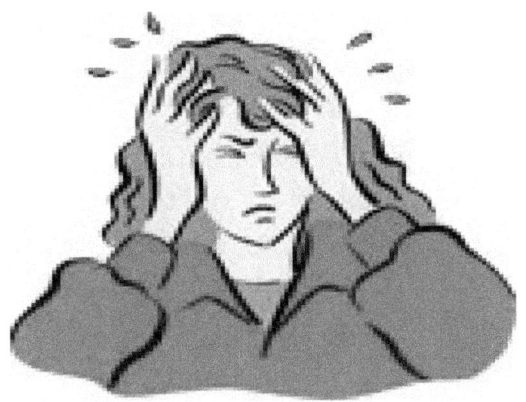

WOMEN AND MOOD SWINGS

When it comes to women mood swings tend to originate purely from hormonal changes. Therefore it is important to pay attention on how to deal with mood swings that occur in women due to hormonal changes.

For some women, the hall ark of the reproductive years is not pregnancy, but rather PMS-specifically the mood-related symptoms.

"Medically speaking, anything that happens just before your period-, for example, spasms, loose bowels, and breast tenderness-is considered premenstrual syndrome," says Steven R. Goldstein, MD, teacher of obstetrics and gynecology at NYU Medical Center in New York City. But for most women it's the mood issues that turn into the characterizing element for what we know as PMS." And, says Goldstein, this can incorporate anything from gentle to direct self-loathing.

Northrup says women who are premenstrual are adept to see remarks made about them as negative, when they are most certainly not. Specialists say that mood swings and different side effects don't fundamentally show anomalous hormone level. "Each study done on women with PMS demonstrates their circling levels of hormones are typical," says Nanette Santoro, Santoro is an executive of the Division of Reproductive Endocrinology at Montefiore Medical Center, and the Albert Einstein College of Medical Center, and the Albert Einstein College of Medicine of New York City. But a few scientists accept that certain hormone metabolites in the brain cause the mood changes-of that a few women simply metabolize hormones differently. Nobody knows without a doubt.

But while doctors may not understand why side effects occur, there are approaches to control them. You can't change your physiology, but you can change your life. Generally when you do that, your hormones react in a good manner.

One of the first lines of protection is to decrease salt intake. Restricting salt will decrease bloating-incorporating water maintenance in the brain. That may ease both physical and emotional symptoms. Removing sugar and constraining caffeine is highly favorable, because both of those chemical can aggravate PMS symptoms.

Chapter 7

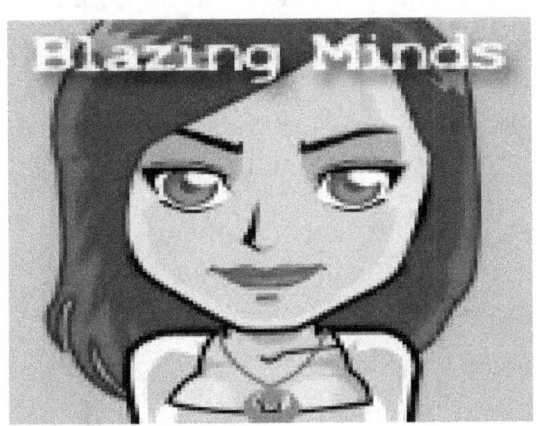

PERIMENOPAUSE MOTHER OF ALL PMS

Keeping in mind medical studies stay sparse, Northrup likewise accepts that women should keep away from eating routine soft drinks and deserts containing aspartame (NutraSweet), and food containing MSG (monosodium glutamate). "Both are stacked with excitotoxins, chemicals that effect cerebrum cells and can exacerbate PMS side effects," she says.

Moreover, it's prescribed that women build the intake of vitamin B6-either by taking supplements, or by including more beans, nuts, vegetable, and fortified bread and oats to your eating routine. Northrup proposes expanding levels of zinc (attempt poultry, fish, nuts, and entire grains, and vegetables).

Lastly, specialists encourage women to give careful consideration to both weight and exercise, and not to take either one to extremes. Keeping up a healthy weight, not overweight, not underweight-and exercising regularly, without trying too hard, serves to simplicity PMS indications, and make them less demanding to adapt to. For extra help, talk with your doctor about conception prevention pills, which can help settle hormone levels. In uncommon occasions, antidepressant prescriptions, for example, Prozac can be utilized a few days a month to help control manifestations.

It can begin in your late 30s, or as late as your late 40s. It's the life change known as perimenopause, a period when egg generation decreases, and hormones can take on a life of their own.

Your conceptive years may appear to be going all out, at the point abruptly; you turn into the mirror image of adolescence. The main thing that happens, is a break in the repetitive way of your menstrual cycle with periods that get to be sporadic-a sign that ovulation is easing off. This can send your hormones on a thrill ride. Each woman imagines that it is the sudden drop in estrogen from not ovulating that causes the issues.

But in actuality, it is the vacillation of estrogen, along with less progesterone, that is behind large portions of the regular manifestations of perimenopause. These manifestations incorporate mood swings and sensitivity, as well as hot flashes, night sweets, and memory issues.

"If you don't get your PMS under control in your 20s and 30s, it will return shouting into your 40s," Northrup says. Perimenopause can be the mother of all PMS assaults. Also, it can last a long time. As demoralizing as this may sound, even the "mother of all PMS" can be controlled. In your 20s and 30s your first line of protection should be dietary changes. If you haven't effectively removed salt, sugars, and white flour, do it now. Furthermore cut back on caffeine and wine. In a few women caffeine and wine can worsen perimenopause manifestations. Furthermore, it is advised that expanding your intake of omega-3 unsaturated fats (found in flax seed, walnut, and eggs), and expanding your calcium intake is favorable in this condition.

Chapter 8

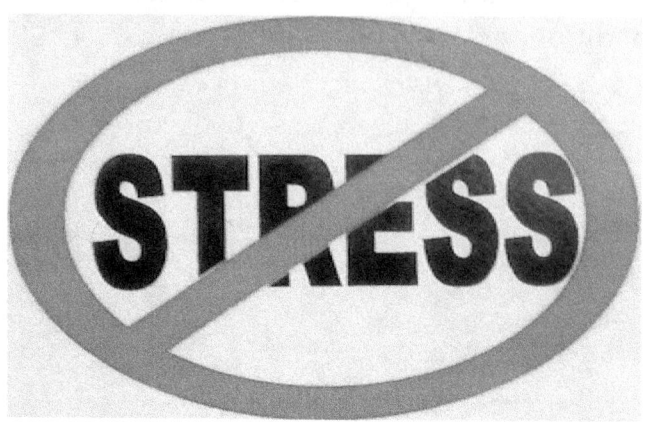

REDUCE STRESS AND MOOD SWINGS

Regarding the matter of your eating schedule, trading basic carbohydrates like bread, pasta and baked good for complex in addition to protein and fiber is favorable to you.

Getting consistent exercise will help in figuring out how to handle stress in a more fortifying manner. It's virtually difficult to decrease stress out of your life, but if you can change the way you handle it-go for a walk, meditate, and listen to music, whatever it is that helps you to release stress-you will see a positive effect on your mood swings.

Described above are the basic tactics you can implement to reduce your stress and mood-swings. It will be positively effective on both yourself and your loved ones. You will be in a calm state of mind and your children will thank you because they need you to be cool headed, and a sensible role model. Following the above described procedures will surely help you to be that for your children.

Mood swings are a natural phenomenon of the human mind. There is no one that is not affected by mood swings. The aim is to avoid any drastic mood swings that might interfere with your day to day life. It's all about learning and practice. If you have the will to control your mood swings, it would greatly affect you, and the people around you in a positive manner.

__Conclusion__

I hope this book was able to help you to manage your mood swings.

The next step is to practice what you just read.

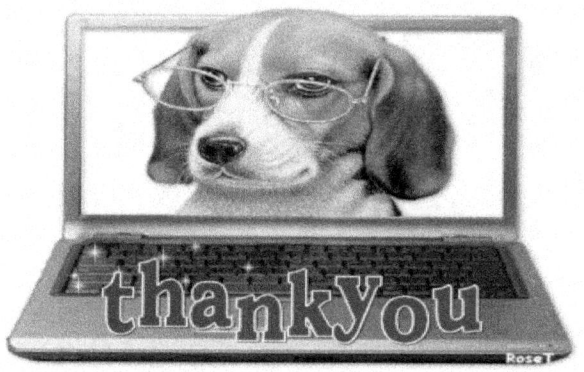

Finally, if you enjoyed this book, would you be kind enough to leave a review for this book on Amazon? It'd be greatly appreciated!

Thank you and good luck!

Preview Of 'Coping with Anxiety Disorder: How to stop anxiety tension.'

Chapter 1

Anxiety is a very common human emotion. However, it can reach at its extreme condition, which is considered as mental illness. It has several negative impacts on body, mind and soul of a person. As a result, that person faces various problems, such as, lack of concentration.

This book is designed to help these individuals. It provides several "Anxiety Tools" to manage and relief from anxiety. These are proven techniques; various researchers, scientists and psychiatrists suggest them. Many of them has been used since the ancient time.

Therefore, do not worry anymore. Start to read this book and eradicate anxiety from your daily life. In addition to that, do not forget to learn them for your future. You can even suggest these tips to your friends and family members.

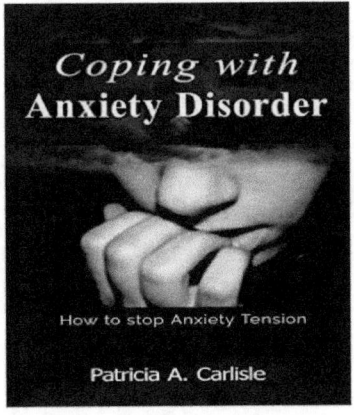

Check out the rest of (Coping with Anxiety Disorders: How to stop Anxiety Tension) on Amazon.com

Check Out My Other Books

Below you'll find some of my other popular books that are popular on Amazon and Kindle as well. Alternatively, you can visit my author page on Amazon to see other work done by me.

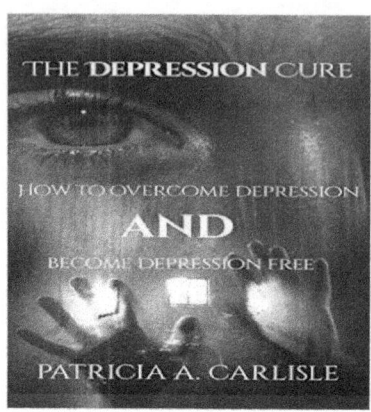

THE DEPRESSION CURE: How to overcome depression and become depression free.

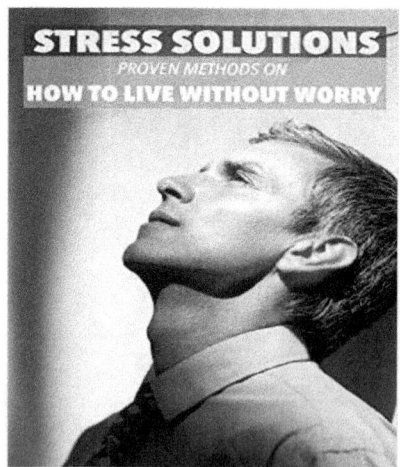

STRESS SOLUTIONS: Proven methods on how to live without worry.

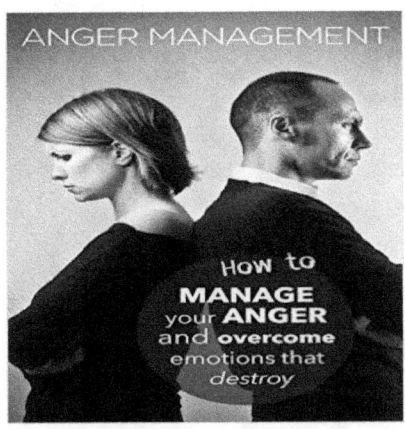

ANGER MANAGEMENT: How to manage your anger and overcome emotions that destroy.

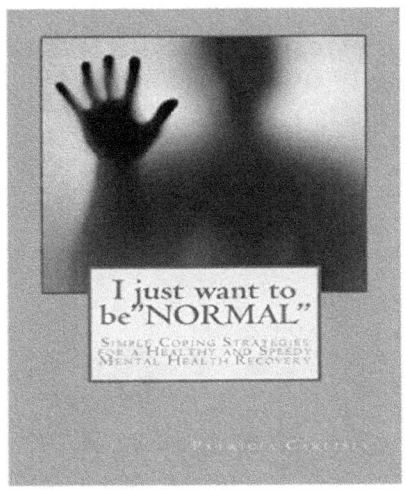

I JUST WANT TO BE "NORMAL" Simple Coping Strategies for a Healthy and Speedy Mental Health Recovery.

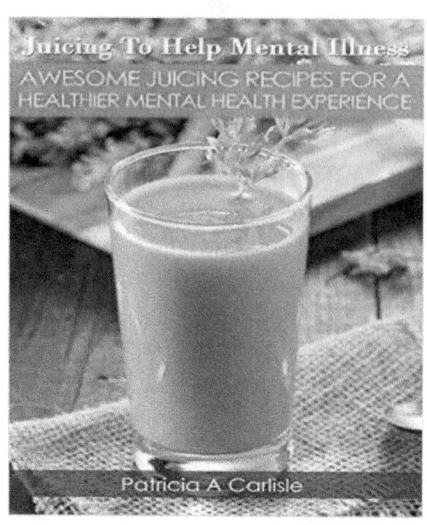

JUICING TO HELP MENTAL ILLNESS: Awesome juicing recipes for a healthier mental health.

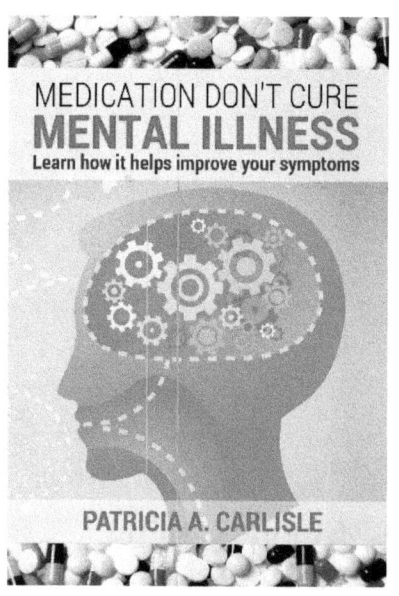

MEDICATION DON'T CURE MENTAL ILLNESS: LEARN HOW IT HELPS IMPROVE YOUR SYMPTOMS.

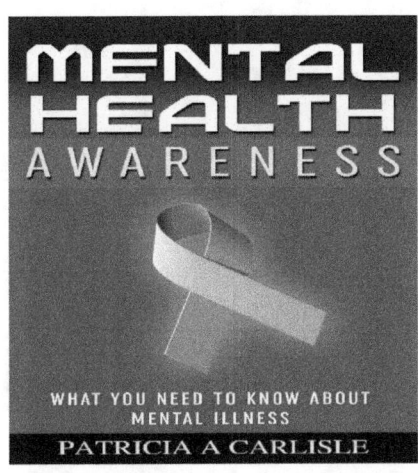

MENTAL HEALTH AWARENESS: WHAT YOU NEED TO KJNOW ABOUT MENTAL ILLNESS

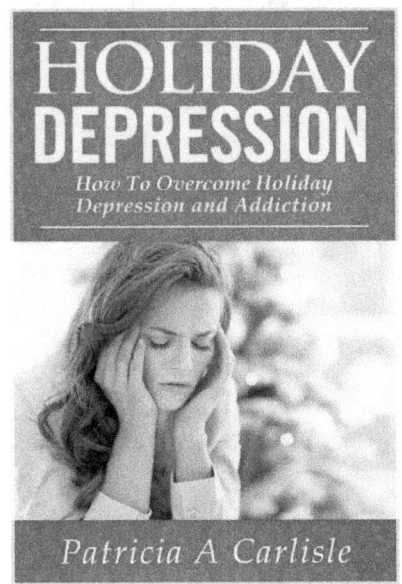

HOLIDAY DEPRESSION: HOW TO OVERCOME HOLIDAY DEPRESSION AND ADDICITON.

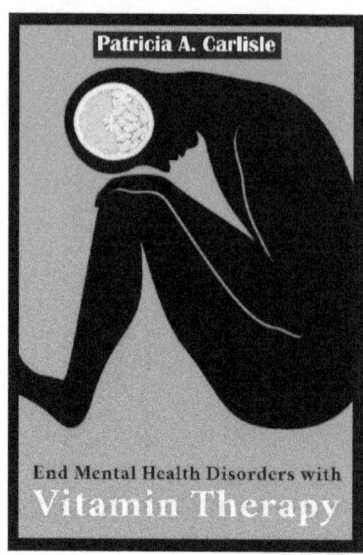

END MENTAL HEALTH DISORDER WITH VITAMIN THERAPY.

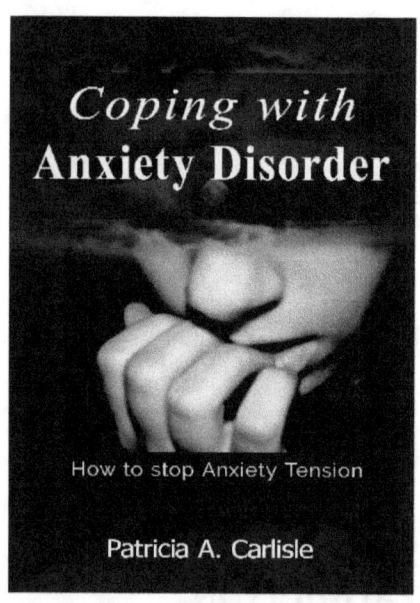

COPING WITH ANXIETY DISORDER: HOW TO STOP ANXIETY TENSION.

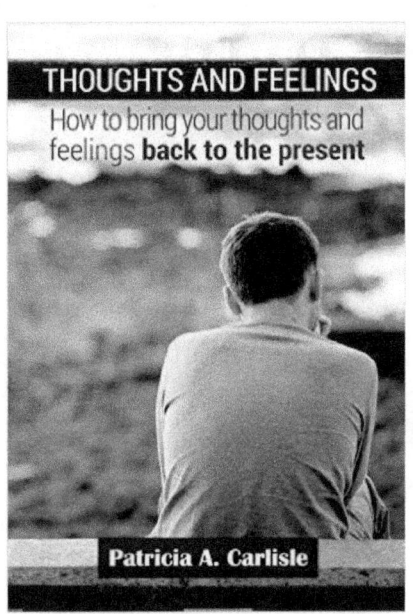

THOUGHTS AND FEELINGS: HOW TO BRING YOUR THOUGHTS AND FEELING BACK TO THE PRESENT.

BONUS: SUBSCRIBE TO THE FREE BOOK

Beginners Guide to Yoga & Meditation

"Stressed out? Do You Feel Like The World Is Crashing Down Around You? Want To Take A Vacation That Will Relax Your Mind, Body And Spirit? Well this Easy To Read Step By Step

E-Book Makes It All Possible!"

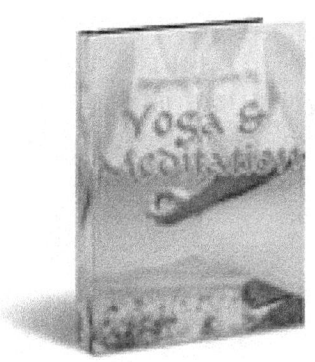

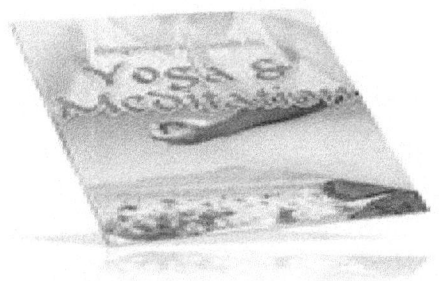

Instructions on how to join our mailing list, and receive a free copy of "Yoga and Meditation" can be found in any of my Kindle eBooks.

NOTE

NOTE

NOTE

NOTE

NOTES